Your Thai

Delicious and Easy Recipes

Tim Singhapat

Table of contents

ASIAN MARINADE 1

Ingredients:

- ¼ cup fish sauce

- ¼ cup soy sauce (if possible low-sodium)

- ½ cup freshly squeezed lime juice

- 1 tablespoon curry powder

- 1 tablespoon light brown sugar

- 1 teaspoon minced garlic Crushed dried red pepper

- 2 tablespoons crispy peanut butter

Directions:

1. Mix all the ingredients in a blender or food processor and pulse until the desired smoothness is achieved.

Yield: Approximately 1¼ cups

ASIAN MARINADE 2

Ingredients:

- ¼ cup chopped green onion
- ¼ cup soy sauce
- ¼ teaspoon ground anise
- ½ cup lime juice
- 1 tablespoon freshly grated gingerroot
- 1 tablespoon honey
- 1 teaspoon Chinese 5-spice powder
- 2 tablespoons hoisin sauce
- 2 tablespoons sesame oil
- 3 cloves garlic, minced
- 3 tablespoons chopped cilantro
- 1 cup vegetable oil

Directions:

1. Mix the lime juice, soy sauce, hoisin sauce, and honey, and blend thoroughly.

2. Slowly whisk in the vegetable and sesame oils. Put in the rest of the ingredients and mix meticulously.

Yield: Approximately 1¼ cups

This recipe has a definite Chinese influence, featuring soy sauce, hoisin sauce, 5-spice powder, and sesame oil

BLACK BEAN PASTE

Ingredients:

- 1 medium to big onion, minced

- 1 tablespoon fish sauce

- 1 teaspoon brown sugar

- 2 cloves garlic, chopped

- 2 jalapeños, seeded and chopped

- 2 tablespoons vegetable oil

- 2 teaspoons lime juice

- 3 green onions, trimmed and cut

- 4 tablespoons canned black beans or black soy beans

Directions:

1. In a moderate-sized-sized sauté pan, heat the oil over moderate-

the onions, jalapeños, garlic, and green onions, and sauté onion becomes translucent.

2. Using a slotted spoon, move the sautéed vegetables to processor or blender (set aside the oil in the sauté pan). rest of the ingredients and process for a short period of time to create a not-paste.

3. Reheat the reserved oil in the sauté pan. Move the paste and heat for five minutes, stirring continuously. If the paste seems thick, add a small amount of water.

Yield: Approximately ½ cup

CHILI TAMARIND PASTE

Ingredients:

- ½ cup dried shrimp

- 1 cup cut shallots

- 1 tablespoon fish sauce

- 1¾ cups vegetable oil, divided

- 12 small Thai chilies or

- 3 tablespoons brown sugar

- 3 tablespoons Tamarind Concentrate (Page 20)

- 6 serrano chilies

- 1 cup garlic

Directions:

1. Put the dried shrimp in a small container. Cover the shrimp stir for a short period of time, and drain; set aside.

2. Pour 1½ cups of the vegetable oil in a moderate-sized deep cooking pan. the oil to roughly 360 degrees on moderate to high heat.

3. Put in the garlic and fry until a golden-brown colour is achieved. Using a slotted move the garlic to a container lined using paper towels.

4. Put in the shallots to the deep cooking pan and fry for two to three minutes; the shallots to the container with the garlic.

5. Fry the reserved shrimp in the deep cooking pan for a couple of minutes; the container.

6. Fry the chilies until they become brittle, approximately half a minute; them to the container. (Allow oil to cool completely discarding.)

7. Mix the fried ingredients, the rest of the oil, and the a food processor; process to make a smooth paste.

8. Put the paste in a small deep cooking pan on moderate heat. Put in the sugar and fish sauce, and cook, stirring once in a while, for approximately five minutes.

9. Allow the paste to return to room temperature before placing in an airtight container.

Yield: Approximately 3 cups

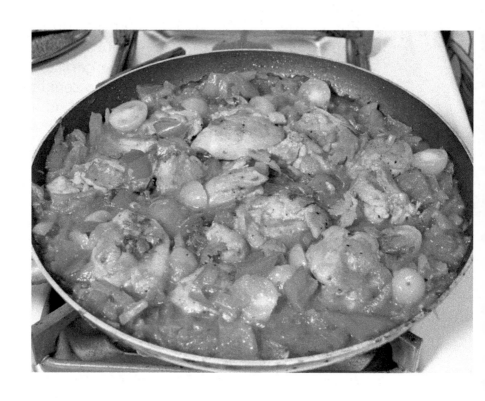

CHILI VINEGAR

Ingredients:

- ½ cup white vinegar

- 2 teaspoons fish sauce

- 3 serrano chilies, seeded and finely cut

Directions:

1. Put all of the ingredients in a container.
2. Allow to sit minimum twenty minutes to allow the flavors to develop.

Yield: Approximately ½ cup

COCONUT MARINADE

Ingredients:

- ¼–½ teaspoon red chili pepper flakes
- 1 tablespoon grated lime zest
- 1 tablespoon minced fresh ginger
- 2 tablespoons shredded, unsweetened coconut
- 2 teaspoons sugar
- 3 tablespoons lime juice
- 3 tablespoons rice wine vinegar
- teaspoon curry powder

Directions:

1. Warm the vinegar using low heat. Put in the coconut and ginger to become tender.
2. Turn off the heat and mix in the rest of the ingredients.

Yield: Approximately ½ cup

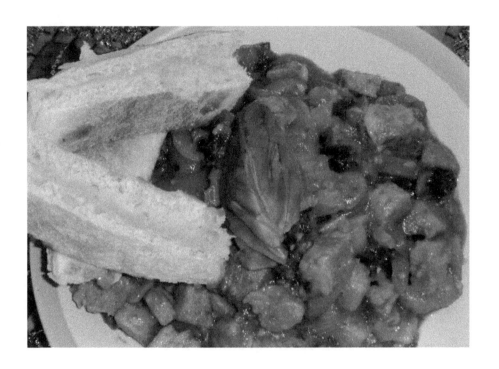

GREEN CURRY PASTE 1

Ingredients:

- ¼ cup vegetable oil

- ½ cup chopped cilantro

- ½ teaspoon ground cloves

- ½ teaspoon shrimp paste

- 1 (1½-inch) piece gingerroot, peeled and chopped

- 1 stalk lemongrass, tough outer leaves removed, inner soft portion chopped

- 1 teaspoon black pepper

- 1 teaspoon ground cumin

- 1 teaspoon salt

- 10 green serrano chilies

- 2 teaspoons grated lime zest

- 2 teaspoons ground coriander

- 2 teaspoons ground nutmeg

- 3 shallots, crudely chopped

- 5 cloves garlic

Directions:

1. Put the first 6 ingredients in a food processor and process mixed. Put in the rest of the ingredients, apart from the vegetable process until the desired smoothness is achieved.

2. Slowly put in the oil until a thick paste May be placed in the fridge up to 4 weeks.

Yield: 1 cup

GREEN CURRY PASTE 2

Ingredients:

- 1 (1-inch) piece ginger, peeled and chopped

- 1 medium onion, chopped

- 1 teaspoon salt

- 1 teaspoon shrimp paste

- 2 green bell peppers, seeded and chopped

- 2 tablespoons vegetable oil

- 2 teaspoons chopped lemongrass

- 2 teaspoons cumin seeds, toasted

- 2–4 green jalapeño chilies,
- 3 cloves garlic, chopped

- 3 tablespoons coriander seeds, toasted

- 3 teaspoons water

- 4 tablespoons chopped cilantro

- 4 tablespoons <u>Tamarind Concentrate (Page 20)</u>

Directions:

1. Put all the ingredients in a food processor and pulse until the desired smoothness is achieved. Move to a small deep cooking pan and bring to a simmer on moderate to low heat. Decrease the heat to low and cook, stirring regularly, for five minutes.

2. Mix in 1 cup of water and bring the mixture to its boiling point. Decrease the heat, cover, and simmer for half an hour

Yield: Approximately 1 cup

LEMON CHILI VINEGAR

Ingredients:

- 1 quart white wine vinegar Peel of 4 limes 8–10 serrano chilies

Directions:

1. Mix all the ingredients in a moderate-sized deep cooking pan and bring to a simmer on moderate heat.

2. Decrease the heat and simmer for about ten minutes.

3. Cool to room temperature, then strain.

Yield: Approximately 1 quart

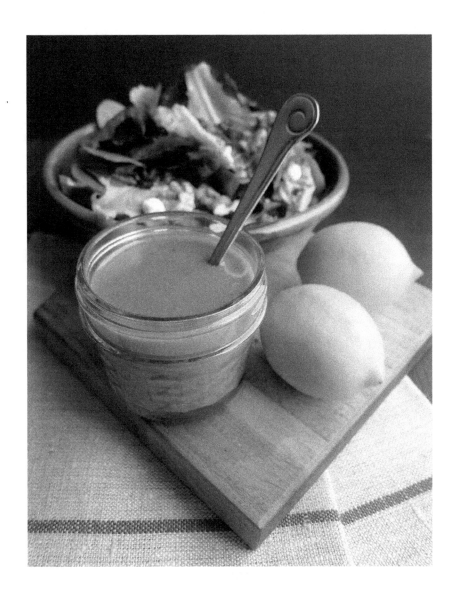

LEMONGRASS MARINADE

Ingredients:

- ¼ tablespoon soy sauce
- 1 cup extra-virgin olive oil
- 1 jalapeño chili pepper, seeded and chopped
- 1 tablespoon fish sauce
- 2 cloves garlic, minced
- 2 stalks lemongrass, trimmed and smashed
- 2 tablespoons chopped cilantro
- 2 tablespoons lime juice

Directions:

1. Pour the olive oil into a pan and heat until warm.
2. Put in the lemongrass and garlic, and cook for a minute. Turn off the heat and let cool completely.
3. Mix in the rest of the ingredients.

Yield: Approximately 1 cups

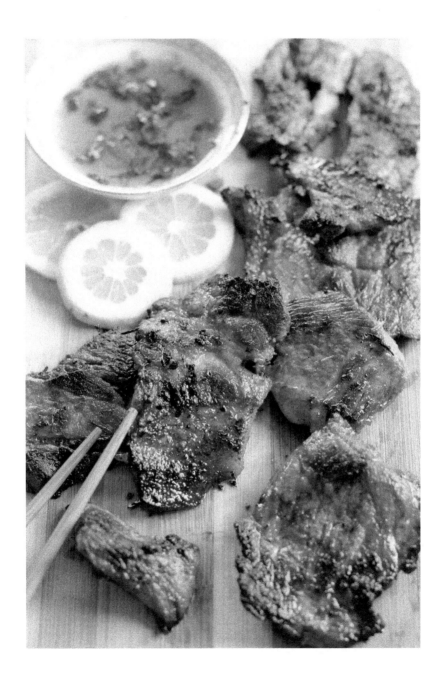

MALAYSIAN MARINADE

Ingredients:

- ¼ cup chopped cilantro
- ¼ cup soy sauce
- ¼ cup vegetable oil
- ½ teaspoon coriander
- ½ teaspoon ground cumin
- 1 green onion, trimmed and thinly cut
- 1 teaspoon grated lime zest
- 2 tablespoons grated gingerroot
- 2 tablespoons honey
- 3 tablespoons lime juice

Directions:

1. Mix the honey, lime juice, lime zest, and soy sauce in a small container.
2. Slowly whisk in the oil.
3. Mix in the rest of the ingredients.

Yield: Approximately 1 cup

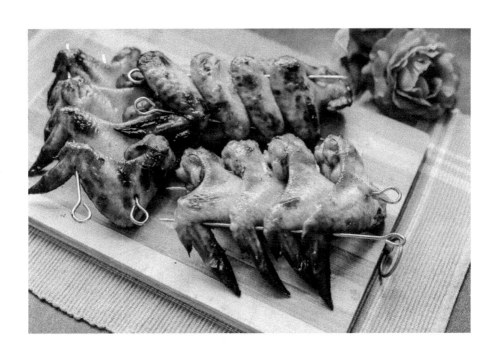

MINTY TAMARIND PASTE

Ingredients:

- ¼ cup peanuts

- ½ cup <u>Tamarind Concentrate (Page 20)</u>

- 1 bunch cilantro leaves

- 1 bunch mint leaves

- 4–5 Thai bird peppers or 2 serrano chilies, seeded and chopped

Directions:

1. Put all the ingredients in a food processor and pulse to make a paste.

Yield: Approximately 2 cups

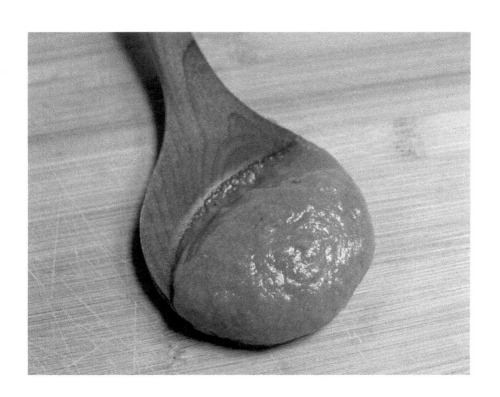

NORTHERN (OR JUNGLE) CURRY PASTE

Ingredients:

- ¼ cup chopped arugula
- ¼ cup chopped chives
- ½ cup chopped mint
- 1 (3-inch) piece ginger, peeled and chopped
- 1 cup chopped basil
- 1 stalk lemongrass, tough outer leaves removed and discarded, inner core minced
- 1 tablespoon shrimp paste
- 12 serrano chilies, seeded and chopped
- 2 tablespoons vegetable oil
- 4 shallots, chopped
- 6–8 Thai bird chilies, seeded and chopped

Directions:

1. In a moderate-sized-sized sauté pan, heat the oil on medium. Put in shrimp paste,

lemongrass, ginger, and shallots, and sauté until shallots start to turn translucent and the mixture is very aromatic.

2. Move the mixture to a food processor and pulse until adding 1 or 2 tablespoons of water to help with the grinding.

3. Put in the rest of the ingredients and more water if required to pulse until crudely mixed.

Yield: Approximately 2 cups

RED CURRY PASTE 1

Ingredients:

- 1 (½-inch) piece ginger, finely chopped

- 1 medium onion, chopped

- 1 stalk lemongrass, outer leaves removed and discarded, inner core finely chopped

- 1 teaspoon salt

- 2 garlic cloves, chopped

- 2 tablespoons Tamarind Concentrate (Page 20)

- 2 teaspoons cumin seeds, toasted

- 2 teaspoons paprika

- 3 kaffir lime leaves or the peel of 1 lime, chopped

- 3 tablespoons coriander seeds, toasted

- 3 tablespoons vegetable oil

- 4 tablespoons water

- 6–8 red serrano chilies, seeded and chopped

Directions:

1. Put all the ingredients in a food processor and pulse until super smooth.

2. Move to a small deep cooking pan and bring to a simmer on moderate to low heat. Decrease the heat to low and cook, stirring regularly, for five minutes.

3. Mix in 1 cup of water and bring the mixture to its boiling point. Decrease the heat, cover, and simmer thirty minutes.

Yield: Approximately ½ cup

RED CURRY PASTE 2

Ingredients:

- 1 (2-inch) piece ginger, peeled and thoroughly minced

- 1 small onion, chopped

- 2 cloves garlic, minced

- 2 stalks lemongrass, tough outer leaves removed and discarded, inner core thoroughly minced

- 2 tablespoons ground turmeric

- 3 big dried red California chilies, seeded and chopped

- 5 dried Thai bird or similar chilies, seeded and chopped

Directions:

1. Put the chilies in a container and cover them with hot water. Allow to stand for minimum 30 minutes. Drain the chilies, saving for later 1 cup of the soaking liquid.

2. Put all the ingredients and 2–3 tablespoons of the soaking liquid in a food processor. Process to make a thick, smooth paste. Put in additional liquid if required.

Yield: Approximately 1 cup

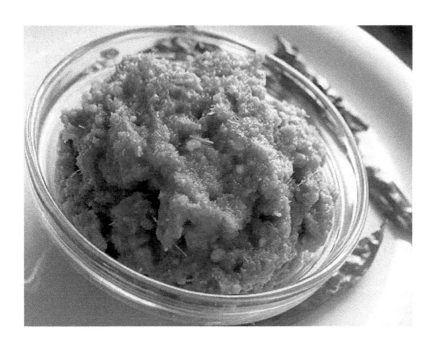

SHREDDED FRESH COCONUT

Ingredients:

1 heavy coconut, with liquid

Directions:

1. Preheat your oven to 400 degrees.

2. Pierce the eye of the coconut using a metal skewer or screwdriver and drain the coconut water (reserve it for later use if you prefer).

3. Bake the coconut for fifteen minutes, then remove and allow to cool.

4. When the coconut is sufficiently cool to handle, use a hammer to break the shell. Using the tip of a knife, cautiously pull the flesh from the shell. Remove any remaining brown membrane with a vegetable peeler.

5. Shred the coconut using a 4-sided grater. Fresh coconut will keep in your fridge for maximum one week.

Yield: Approximately 1 cup

SOUTHERN (OR MASSAMAN) CURRY PASTE

Ingredients:

- ¼ teaspoon ground cinnamon

- ¼ teaspoon whole black peppercorns

- ½ teaspoon cardamom seeds, toasted

- 1 (1-inch) piece ginger, peeled and minced

- 1 stalk lemongrass, tough outer leaves removed and discarded, inner core finely chopped

- 1 teaspoon lime peel

- 1 teaspoon salt

- 1 teaspoon shrimp paste (not necessary)

- 2 tablespoons coriander seeds, toasted

- 2 tablespoons vegetable oil

- 2 teaspoons brown sugar

- 2 teaspoons cumin seeds, toasted

- 2 whole cloves

- 3 tablespoons <u>Tamarind Concentrate (Page 20)</u>

- 3 tablespoons water

- 6–8 big dried red chilies (often called California chilies), soaked in hot water for five minutes and drained

Directions:

1. Put all ingredients in a food processor and pulse until the desired smoothness is achieved.

2. Move to a small deep cooking pan and bring to a simmer on moderate to low heat. Decrease the heat to low and cook, stirring regularly, for five minutes.

3. Mix in 1 cup of water and bring the mixture to its boiling point. Decrease the heat, cover, and simmer thirty minutes.

Yield: Approximately 1 cup

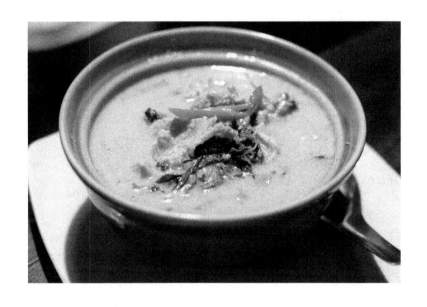

TAMARIND CONCENTRATE

Ingredients:

- 1 cup warm water

- 2 ounces seedless tamarind pulp (sold in Asian markets)

Directions:

1. Put the tamarind pulp and water in a small container for about twenty minutes or until the pulp is tender.

2. Break the pulp apart using the backside of a spoon and stir until blended.

3. Pour the mixture through a fine-mesh sieve, pushing the tender pulp through the strainer. Discard any fibrous pulp remaining in the strainer.

Yield: Approximately 1 cup

TAMARIND MARINADE

Ingredients:

- ¼ cup fresh lime juice

- ¼ cup toasted, unsweetened coconut

- ¼ cup vegetable oil

- ½ cup chopped cilantro leaves

- 1 shallot, chopped

- 1 tablespoon brown sugar

- 1 tablespoon diced fresh gingerroot

- 1 tablespoon soy sauce

- 1½ cups Tamarind Concentrate (Page 20)

- 2 garlic cloves, minced

- 4 pieces lime peel (roughly ½-inch by two-inches)

Directions:

1. Mix the tamarind and lime peel in a small deep cooking pan and bring to a simmer; cook for five minutes.

2. Turn off the heat and cool completely. Mix in the rest of the ingredients.

Yield: Approximately 2 cups

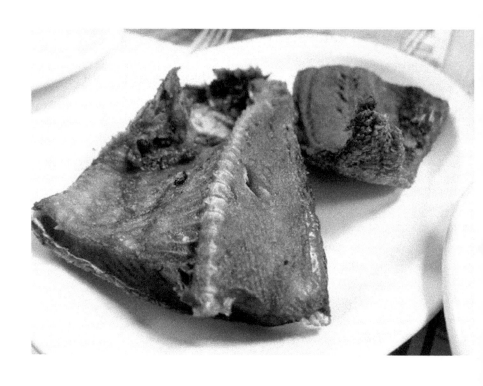

THAI GRILLING RUB

Ingredients:

- 1 teaspoon dried lime peel

- 1 teaspoon freshly ground black pepper

- 1 teaspoon ground ginger
-
  4 teaspoons salt

Directions:

1. Mix all the ingredients and mix meticulously. Store in an airtight container.

2. To use, wash the meat of your choice under cool water and pat dry; drizzle the meat with the spice mixture (to taste) and rub it in together with some olive oil, then grill or broil to your preference.

Yield: Approximately

THAI MARINADE 1

Ingredients:

- ¼ cup chopped cilantro
- ¼ cup fresh lime juice
- ¼ teaspoon hot pepper flakes
- ½ cup sesame oil
- 1 big stalk lemongrass, crushed
- 1 tablespoon brown sugar
- 2 tablespoons chopped peanuts
- 2 tablespoons fish sauce
- 3 cloves garlic, minced

Directions:

1. Mix the fish sauce and lime juice in a small container.
2. Slowly whisk in the sesame oil, then mix in rest of the ingredients.

Yield: Approximately 1 cup

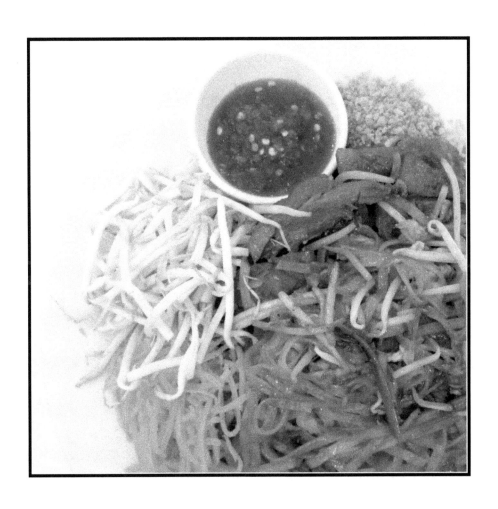

THAI MARINADE 2

Ingredients:

- ¼ cup chopped basil leaves

- ¼ cup chopped mint leaves

- ¼ cup peanut oil

- ½ cup rice wine

- 1 small onion, chopped

- 1 tablespoon chopped gingerroot

- 1 tablespoon sweet soy sauce

- 2 tablespoons chopped lemongrass

- 3 cloves garlic, minced

- 3 tablespoons fish sauce

Directions:

1. Mix the fish sauce, sweet soy sauce, and the rice wine in a small container.

2. Slowly whisk in the peanut oil, then mix in rest of the ingredients.

Yield: Approximately 1½ cups

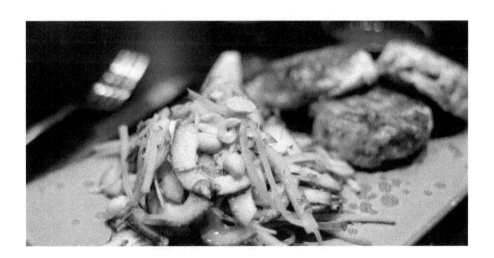

THAI MARINADE 3

Ingredients:

- ¼ cup chopped cilantro leaves

- ¼ cup lime juice

- ½ cup Red Curry Paste (Page 17)

- 1 (12-ounce) can coconut milk

- 1 stalk lemongrass, roughly chopped

- 1 tablespoon sweet soy sauce

- 1 teaspoon fresh gingerroot, chopped

- 2 tablespoons fish sauce

- 6 kaffir lime leaves, finely cut

Directions:

1. Mix the coconut milk, curry paste, lemongrass, and kaffir leaves in a small deep cooking pan; bring to a simmer on moderate heat.

2. Decrease the heat and carry on simmering for fifteen minutes.

3. Turn off the heat and let cool to room temperature.

Yield: Approximately 2 cups

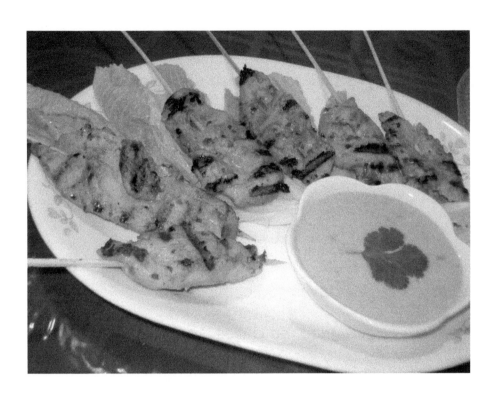

THAI VINEGAR MARINADE

Ingredients:

- ¼ cup chopped lemongrass

- 1 tablespoon fresh grated gingerroot

- 1 tablespoon sugar

- 2–3 tablespoons vegetable oil

- 3 tablespoons chopped green onion

- 3½ cups rice wine vinegar

- 4 cloves garlic, minced

- 6 dried red chilies, seeded and crumbled

Directions:

1. Put the garlic, chilies, green onions, and ginger in a food processor or blender and process to make a paste.

2. Heat the oil in a wok or frying pan, put in the paste, and stir-fry for four to five minutes. Turn off the heat and allow the mixture to cool completely.

3. In a small deep cooking pan, bring the vinegar to its boiling point. Put in the sugar and the lemongrass; decrease the heat and simmer for about twenty minutes.

4. Mix in the reserved paste.

Yield: Approximately 3 cups

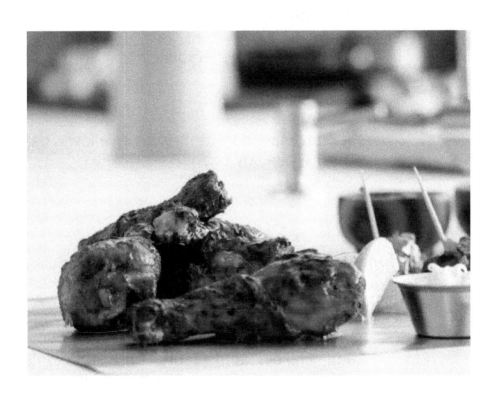

YELLOW BEAN SAUCE

Ingredients:

- 1 (½-inch) piece ginger, peeled and chopped

- 1 medium to big onion, minced

- 1 teaspoon ground coriander

- 2 serrano chilies, seeded and chopped

- 2 tablespoons lime juice

- 2 tablespoons vegetable oil

- 2 tablespoons water

- 4 tablespoons fermented yellow beans (fermented soy beans)

Directions:

1. In a moderate-sized-sized sauté pan, heat the oil on moderate heat. Put in the onion and chilies, and sauté until the onion becomes translucent. Mix in the ginger and coriander, and carry on cooking for half a minute.

2. Put in the beans, lime juice, and water, and simmer using low heat for about ten minutes.

3. Move the mixture to a blender and process until the desired smoothness is achieved.

Yield: Approximately 1 cup

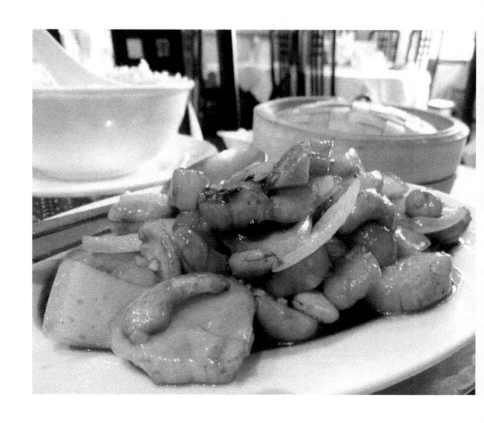

5 MINUTE DIPPING SAUCE

Ingredients:

- ½ teaspoon dried red pepper flakes

- 1 tablespoon fish sauce

- 1 tablespoon lime juice

- 1 teaspoon minced fresh ginger

- 1 teaspoon sugar

Directions:

1. In a small container, dissolve the sugar in 1 tablespoon of water.

2. Mix in the rest of the ingredients; tweak seasonings if required. Serve at room temperature.

Yield: Approximately 4 tablespoons

BANANA, TAMARIND, AND MINT SALSA

Ingredients:

- ¼ cup <u>Tamarind Concentrate (Page 20)</u>

- 1 roasted red jalapeño, seeded and chopped

- 1 tablespoon chopped fresh mint

- 1 tablespoon lime juice

- 1 teaspoon brown sugar
- 4 ripe bananas, peeled and finely diced

Directions:

1. Lightly fold all the ingredients together.

Yield: Approximately 2 cups

This unique salsa goes perfectly with roasted or grilled poultry or game.

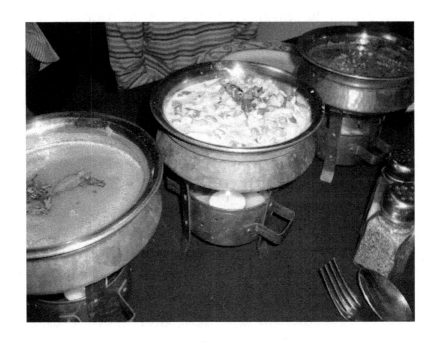

GINGER-LEMONGRASS VINAIGRETTE

Ingredients:

- ¼ cup grated fresh gingerroot

- 1 quart rice wine vinegar

- 2 stalks lemongrass, outer leaves removed and discarded, inner core slightly mashed

Directions:

1. Mix all the ingredients in a nonreactive pot and simmer using low heat for half an hour.

2. Turn off the heat and allow it to stand overnight. Strain before you serve.

Yield: Approximately 1 quart

JALAPEÑO-LIME VINAIGRETTE

Ingredients:

- 1 cup vegetable or canola oil

- 1 jalapeño, seeded and chopped

- 1 tablespoon sugar

- 1 cup lime juice

- Salt and pepper to taste

Directions:

1. Put the jalapeño, lime juice, sugar, and salt and pepper in a food processor; blend for a minute.

2. While continuing to blend, slowly put in the oil; blend for half a minute or until well blended.

Yield: Approximately 1 cups

MANGO-CUCUMBER SALSA

Ingredients:

- ¼ cup cut green onion

- ¼ cup orange juice

- 1 firm, ripe mango, peeled, seeded, and slice into ¼-inch dice

- 1 medium cucumber, seeded and slice into ¼-inch dice

- 1 teaspoon vegetable oil

- 2 teaspoons lime juice

- Salt and pepper to taste

Directions:

1. Mix all the ingredients in a small container.

Yield: Approximately 2 cups

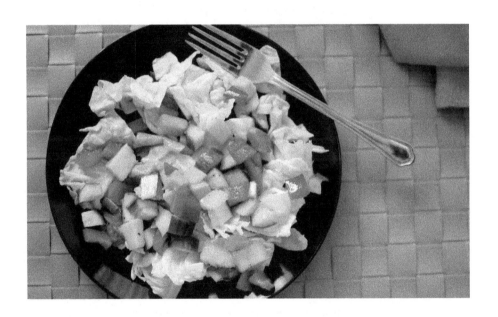

MANGO-PINEAPPLE SALSA

Ingredients:

- ¼ cup snipped chives

- ½ cup diced red onion

- 1 cup diced pineapple

  1 cup mango pieces
- 1 cup seeded and chopped tomato

- 1 serrano chili, seeded and chopped

- 2 tablespoons lime juice

  2 tablespoons vegetable oil Salt and pepper
- to taste

- 3 tablespoons chopped cilantro

Directions:

1. Mix all the ingredients in a small container.
2. Cover and place in your fridge for minimum 2 hours before you serve.

Yield: Approximately 4 cups

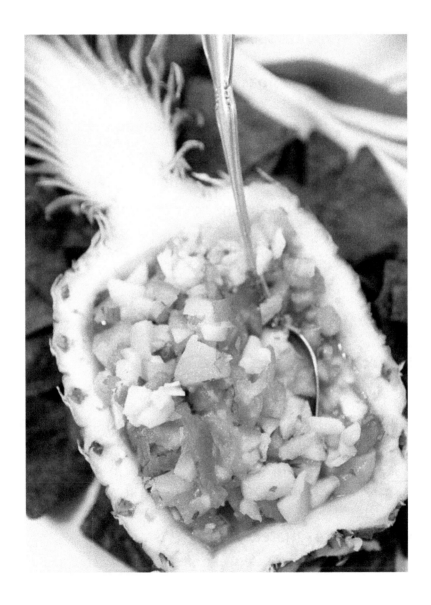

MINT-CILANTRO "CHUTNEY"

Ingredients:

- ½ teaspoon minced honey
- ¾ cup packed cilantro
- ¾ cup packed mint leaves
- 2 teaspoons honey
- 3 tablespoons sour cream
- 1 cup unsalted peanuts, toasted
- Salt and pepper to taste

Directions:

1. Put the peanuts in a food processor and finely grind.
2. Put in the rest of the ingredients to the processor and blend until well blended.

Yield: Approximately 2 cups

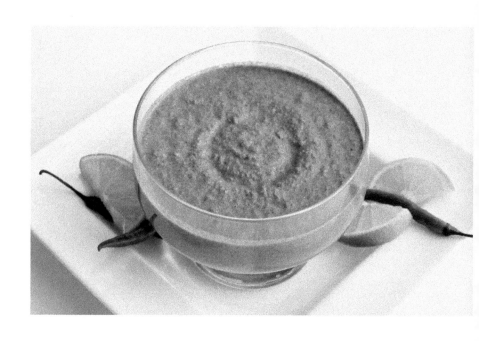

MINTY DIPPING SAUCE

Ingredients:

- ¼ cup chopped mint leaves
- ¼ cup lime juice
- 1 serrano chili, seeded and diced
- 1 tablespoon grated lime zest
- 2 cloves garlic, minced
- 2 tablespoons fish sauce

Directions:

1. Put all the ingredients in a blender and process until the desired smoothness is achieved.
2. Serve with a variety of grilled, skewered meats and raw or blanched vegetables.

Yield: Approximately 1 cup

PEANUT DIPPING SAUCE 1

Ingredients:

- ¼ cup chicken or vegetable stock

- ¼ cup heavy cream

- ¼ cup lemon juice

- 1 teaspoon grated gingerroot

- 1½ cups coconut milk

- 2 tablespoons brown sugar

- 2 tablespoons soy sauce

- 3–4 dashes (or to taste) Tabasco

- 4 cloves garlic, pressed

- 1 cup crispy peanut butter

Directions:

1. Mix the peanut butter, coconut milk, lemon juice, soy sauce, brown sugar, ginger, garlic, and Tabasco in a small deep cooking pan on moderate heat. Cook while stirring

continuously, until the sauce has the consistency of heavy cream, approximately fifteen minutes.

2. Move the mixture to a blender and purée for a short period of time.

3. Put in the stock and cream, and blend until the desired smoothness is achieved.

Yield: Approximately 2 cups

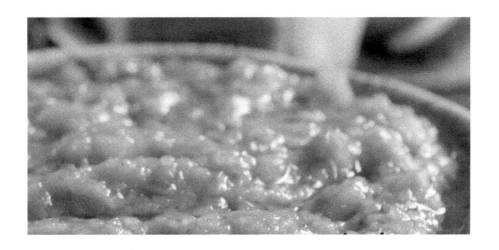

PEANUT DIPPING SAUCE 2

Ingredients:

- ¼ cup fresh lime juice

- ¼ cup half-and-half or heavy cream

- ¼ cup low-sodium beef broth

- 1 teaspoon grated gingerroot

- 1½ cups unsweetened canned coconut milk 2 tablespoons brown sugar 2 tablespoons soy sauce

- 2 teaspoons minced garlic Ground cayenne or crushed red pepper flakes to taste

- 1 cup crispy peanut butter

Directions:

1. In a moderate-sized-sized deep cooking pan, mix the peanut butter, coconut milk, lime juice, soy sauce, brown sugar, ginger, garlic, and cayenne.

2. Stirring continuously, cook on moderate heat until the sauce thickens, approximately fifteen minutes.

3. Take away the sauce from the heat and put in the beef broth and cream. Using a hand mixer, blend until the desired smoothness is achieved. Heat for a short period of time just prior to serving.

Yield: Approximately 2 cups

PEANUT DIPPING SAUCE 3

Ingredients:

- ½ cup smooth peanut butter

- 1 cup canned coconut milk

- 1 tablespoon fish sauce

- 1 teaspoon fresh lemon juice

- 1 teaspoon Tabasco

- 2 tablespoons fresh lime juice

- 2 teaspoons light brown sugar

- 2 teaspoons soy sauce

- 3 shallots

Directions:

1. Roast the shallots in an oven preheated to 325 degrees for approximately five minutes or until tender. Allow them to cool to roughly room temperature.

2. Put all ingredients in a blender or food processor and pulse until the desired smoothness is achieved.

Yield: Approximately 2 cups

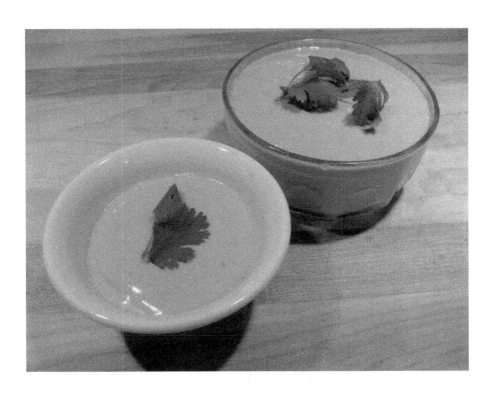

PEANUT PESTO

Ingredients:

¼ cup honey

¼ teaspoon (or to taste) red pepper flakes ½ cup sesame oil

½ cup soy sauce

1 cup unsalted roasted peanuts

2–3 cloves garlic, minced

1 cup water

Directions:

1. Put the peanuts in a food processor fitted using a metal blade; pulse until fine.
2. While continuing to blend, put in the rest of the ingredients one by one through the feed tube until well mixed.

Yield: Approximately 2 cups

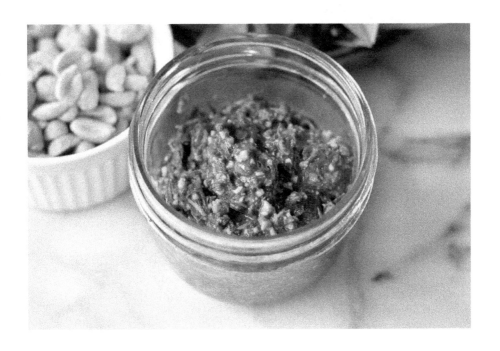

QUICK HOT DIPPING SAUCE

Ingredients:

- ½ cup white vinegar

- 1 loaded tablespoon prepared chili-garlic sauce

Directions:

1. Mix the 2 ingredients before you serve.

Yield: Approximately ½ cup

SPICY THAI DRESSING

Ingredients:

- 1 fresh red cayenne pepper or

- 1 tablespoon plus 1 teaspoon rice wine vinegar

- 1 tablespoon sesame oil

- 1 teaspoon grated gingerroot

- 1 teaspoon sugar

- 2 cloves garlic

- 2 tablespoons soy sauce

- 2 Thai peppers, stemmed, seeded, and slice into pieces

- 3 tablespoons water

Directions:

1. Put all the ingredients in a blender and process until the desired smoothness is achieved.

Yield: Approximately 1 cup

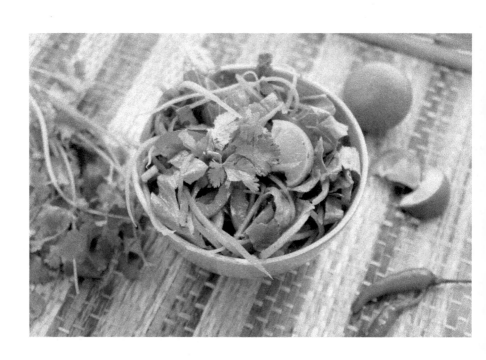

SWEET-AND-SOUR DIPPING SAUCE

Ingredients:

- ½ cup white vinegar

- ½ teaspoon salt

- 1 cup sugar

- 1 loaded tablespoon prepared chili-garlic sauce

Directions:

1. Mix the vinegar, sugar, and salt in a small deep cooking pan on moderate to high heat; bring to its boiling point, reduce to a simmer, and cook for eight to ten minutes, stirring once in a while.

2. Mix in the chili sauce and turn off the heat. Allow to cool to room temperature before you serve.

Yield: Approximately 1½ cups

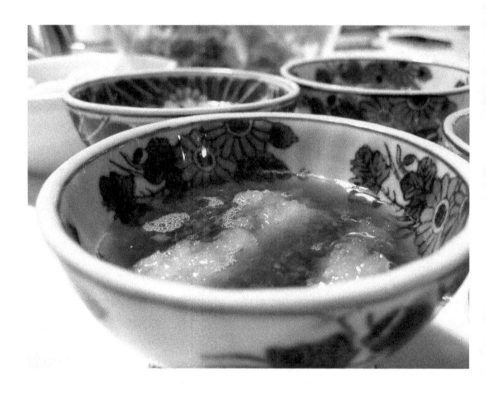

THAI-STYLE PLUM DIPPING SAUCE

Ingredients:

- 2 tablespoons honey Tabasco to taste

- 1 cup plum preserves

- 1 cup water

- 1 cup white vinegar

Directions:

1. Put all the ingredients apart from the Tabasco in a food processor or blender, and process until the desired smoothness is achieved.

2. Move the mixture to a small deep cooking pan and bring to its boiling point on moderate heat; decrease the heat and simmer until thick, approximately twelve to fifteen minutes.

3. Allow to cool completely, then mix in the Tabasco.

Yield: Approximately 2 cups

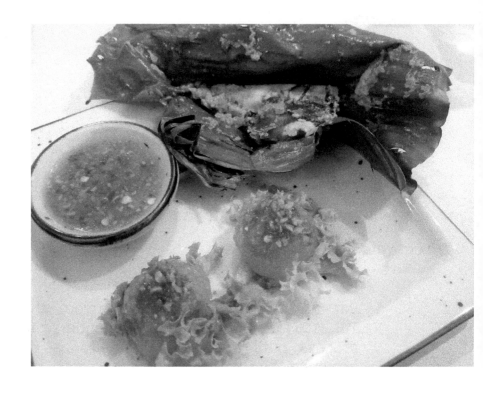

3 FLAVOR RICE STICKS

Ingredients:

- 1 pound rice sticks, broken into 3-inch segments
- Cayenne pepper to taste
- Curry powder to taste
- Salt to taste
- Vegetable oil for frying

Directions:

1. Pour 2 to 3 inches of vegetable oil into a big frying pan and heat to 350 degrees. Fry the rice sticks in batches (ensuring not to overcrowd the pan), turning them swiftly as they puff up. After they stop crackling in the oil, move the puffed sticks to paper towels to drain.

2. While the rice sticks are still hot, drizzle salt on 1 batch; drizzle a second batch with curry powder; and a third batch with cayenne pepper to taste.

Yield: Servings 4–6

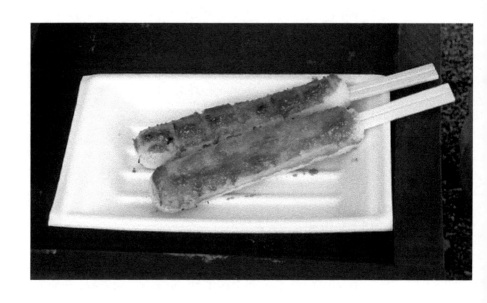

BASIL AND SHRIMP WEDGES

Ingredients:

- ½ cup julienned basil

- ½ pound cooked salad shrimp

- 1 green onion, trimmed and thinly cut

  1 teaspoon fish sauce
- 1½ teaspoons vegetable oil, divided

- 2 tablespoons water

- 4 eggs

- Salt and pepper to taste

Directions:

1. Put 1 teaspoon of the vegetable oil in a sauté pan on moderate heat. Put in the shrimp and green onion, and sauté until the shrimp are warmed through, roughly two minutes. Put in the basil and fish sauce and cook for 1 more minute. Set aside.

2. In a big container, whisk together the eggs, water, and salt and pepper, then mix in the shrimp mixture.

3. Put the remaining ½ teaspoon of vegetable oil in an omelet pan on moderate heat. Put in the egg mixture and cook until the omelet starts to brown. Turn over the omelet and carry on cooking until set.

4. To serve, slide the omelet onto a serving plate and cut it into wedges. Serve with a Thai dipping sauce of your choice.

Yield: Servings 4–6 as an appetizer or 2 as a brunch item

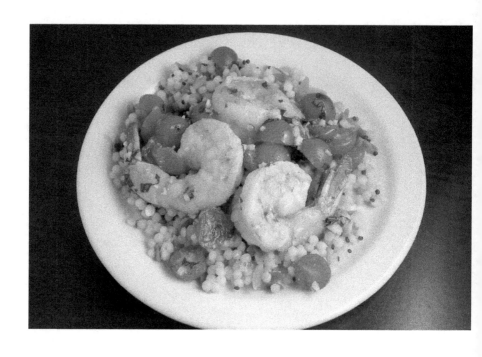

CHICKEN, SHRIMP, AND BEEF SATAY
Chicken

- 1 recipe Peanut Dipping Sauce

- 1 recipe Thai Marinade (Page 22)

- 3 whole boneless, skinless chicken breasts, cut into lengthy strips about ½-inch wide

Directions:

Thread the chicken strips onto presoaked bamboo skewers or onto metal skewers. Put the skewers in a flat pan and cover with marinade. Marinate the chicken in your fridge overnight.

2. Cook the skewers on the grill or under the broiler, coating and turning them until they are thoroughly cooked, approximately six to eight minutes.
3. Serve with the peanut sauce for dipping.

Shrimp

- 1 recipe Peanut Dipping Sauce

- 1 recipe Thai Marinade (Page 22)

- 24 big shrimp, shelled and deveined

Directions:

1. Thread the shrimp onto presoaked bamboo skewers or onto metal skewers (about 3 shrimp per skewer). Put the skewers in a flat pan and cover with marinade. Marinate the shrimp for minimum fifteen minutes, but no longer than an hour.

2. Cook the skewers on the grill or under the broiler, coating and turning them frequently until just opaque, approximately three to four minutes.

3. Serve with the peanut sauce for dipping.

Yield: 4–6 chicken skewers or 6–8 shrimp or beef skewers

Beef

- 1 recipe Thai Marinade (Page 22)

- 1 recipe Peanut Dipping Sauce

- 1-1½ pounds sirloin steak, fat and sinew removed, cut into ½-inch-wide strips

Directions:

1. Thread the beef strips onto presoaked bamboo skewers or onto metal skewers. Put the skewers in a flat pan and cover with marinade. Marinate the beef in your fridge overnight.
2. Cook the skewers on the grill or under the broiler, coating and turning them frequently until done to your preference, approximately six to eight minutes for medium.

3. Serve with the peanut sauce for dipping.

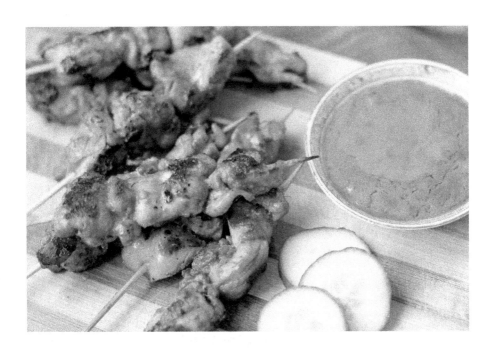

CHINESE-STYLE DUMPLINGS

Ingredients:

- ¼ cup sticky rice flour

- ¼ cup tapioca flour

- ½ cup water

- 1 cup rice flour

- 1 tablespoon soy sauce

- 1 teaspoon vegetable oil

- 2 cups chives, cut into ½–inch lengths

Directions:

1. In a moderate-sized-sized deep cooking pan, mix together the sticky rice flour, the rice flour, and the water. Turn the heat to moderate and cook, stirring continuously until the mixture has the consistency of glue. (If the mixture becomes too sticky, decrease the heat to low.) Take away the batter from the heat and swiftly mix in the tapioca flour. Set aside to cool completely.

2. In the meantime, put in the vegetable oil to a frying pan big enough to easily hold the chives, and heat on high. Put in the chives and the soy sauce. Stir-fry the chives just until they wilt. Be careful not to let the chives cook excessively. Turn off the heat and save for later.

3. Once the dough has reached room temperature, check its consistency. If it is too sticky to work with, add a little extra tapioca flour.

4. To make the dumplings, roll the batter into balls an inch in diameter. Using your fingers, flatten each ball into a disk
approximately four inches across. Ladle approximately 1 tablespoon of the chives into the middle of each disk. Fold the disk in half and pinch the edges together to make a halfmoon-shaped packet.

5. Put the dumplings in a prepared steamer for five to 8 minutes or until the dough is cooked. Serve with a spicy dipping sauce of your choice.

Yield: 15–20 dumplings

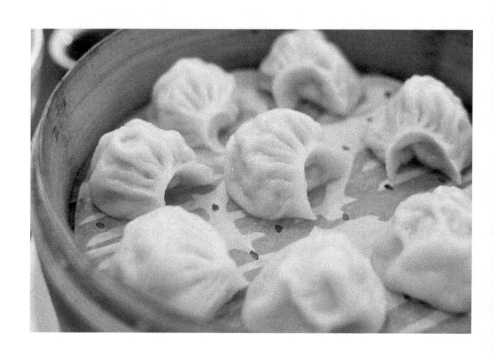

COLD SESAME NOODLES

Ingredients:

- ¼ cup creamy peanut butter or tahini

- ¼–½ teaspoon dried red pepper flakes

- 1 pound angel hair pasta

- 1 tablespoon grated ginger

- 1–2 green onions, trimmed and thinly cut (not necessary)

- 2 tablespoons rice vinegar

- 2 tablespoons sesame oil

Directions:

1. Cook the pasta in accordance with package directions. Wash under cold water, then set aside.

2. Vigorously whisk together the rest of the ingredients; pour over pasta, tossing to coat.

3. Decorate using green onion if you wish.

Yield: Servings 2–4

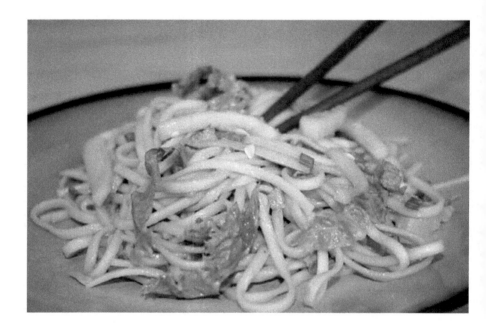

CRAB SPRING ROLLS

Ingredients:

- ¼–½ teaspoon grated lime peel

- 1 pound crabmeat, picked over to remove any shells, and shredded

- 1 tablespoon mayonnaise

- 2 egg yolks, lightly beaten

- Canola oil for deep frying

- fifteen small, soft Boston lettuce leaves

- fifteen spring roll or egg roll wrappers

- Mint leaves

- Parsley leaves

Directions:

1. In a small container, combine the crabmeat with the mayonnaise and lime peel.

2. Put 1 tablespoon of the crabmeat mixture in the middle of 1 spring roll wrapper. Fold a pointed end of the wrapper over the crabmeat, then fold the opposite point over the top of the folded point. Brush a small amount of the egg yolk over the top of the uncovered wrapper, then fold the bottom point over the crabmeat and roll to make a tight packet; set aside. Repeat with the rest of the crabmeat and wrappers.

3. Heat the oil to 365 degrees in a frying pan or deep fryer. Deep-fry the rolls three to 4 at a time for a couple of minutes or so, until they are a golden brown; drain using paper towels.

4. To serve, wrap each spring roll in a wrapper with a single piece of lettuce, and a drizzling of mint and parsley. Serve with a dipping sauce of your choice.

Yield: fifteen rolls

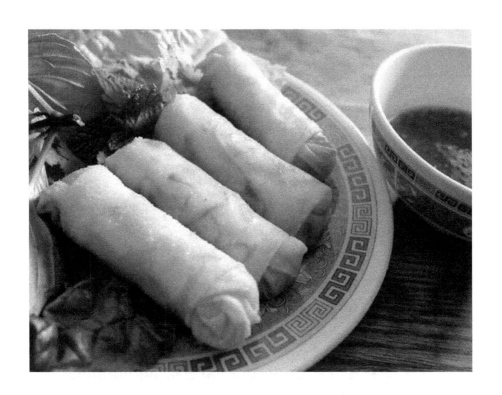

CRISPY MUSSEL PANCAKES

Ingredients:

- ¼ cup all-purpose flour

- ¼ teaspoon salt

- ½ cup tapioca flour

- ¾ cup water

- 1 cup shelled mussels (approximately 1 pound before shelling)

- 1 teaspoon baking powder

- 2 cups bean sprouts

- 2 tablespoons chopped cilantro, plus extra for decoration Salt and ground
- pepper to taste

Directions:

1. To prepare the mussels, wash them swiftly using cool running water. Debeard the

mussels by pulling out the brown membrane that is sometimes still attached. Discard any mussels that are already open. Fill a big frying pan with ½ to an inch of water. Bring the water to its boiling point, then put in the mussels, cover, and allow to steam approximately four minutes or until the mussels have opened, shaking the pan every so frequently. Drain the mussels through a colander. Allow to cool to room temperature and then use a small fork to pull the meat from the shell; set aside using paper towels.

2. In a moderate-sized-sized mixing container, mix together the flours, the salt, and the baking powder. Whisk in the water to make a thin batter.

3. Preheat your oven to 200 degrees. In a large, heavy-bottomed frying pan, heat the vegetable oil on moderate to high heat. Pour half of the batter into the frying pan and top with half of the mussels. Cook until the batter has set and turned golden, approximately 2 minutes. Cautiously flip the pancake over and carry on cooking until golden. Take away the pancake to a baking sheet lined with some foil and place it in your oven to keep warm. Repeat to make a second pancake with the rest of the batter and mussels.

4. Put in 1 teaspoon of vegetable oil to the frying pan if it is dry, and raise the heat to high. Put in the bean sprouts, drizzle with salt and ground pepper to taste, and stir-fry swiftly just to heat

through, approximately half a minute.

5. To serve, place each pancake in the middle of a plate. Top with the bean sprouts, some cilantro, and a grind of fresh pepper. Serve with a sweet-and-sour sauce of your choice.

Yield: Servings 2–4

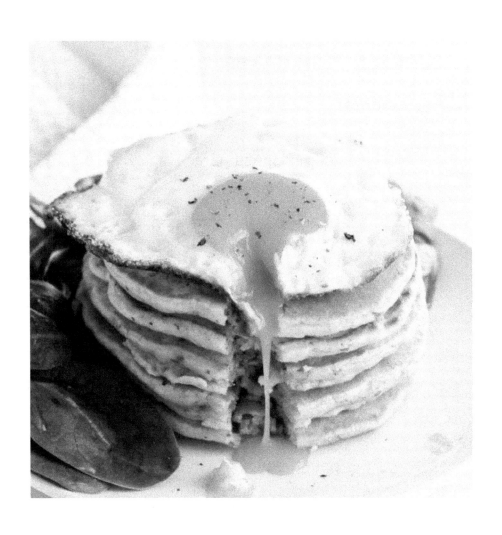

CURRIED FISH CAKES

Ingredients:

- ¼ cup chopped garlic

- ¼ cup chopped lemongrass, inner portion only ¼ cup chopped
- shallots

- ½ pound French beans, trimmed and finely chopped ½
- tablespoon salt

- ½ teaspoon peppercorns

- 1 egg, beaten

- 1 pound boneless whitefish steak, minced

- 1 tablespoon chopped ginger

- 1 tablespoon shrimp paste

- 1 teaspoon grated lime peel

- 5–10 dried chilies, seeded, soaked, and shredded
- Vegetable oil for frying

Directions:

1. Put the shallots, garlic, lemongrass, ginger, peppercorns, lime peel, shrimp paste, chilies, and salt in a food processor or blender and process to make a smooth paste.

2. Put in the fish to the food processor and pulse until well blended with the spice paste. Put in the beaten egg and mix one more time. Move the fish mixture to a big mixing container and mix in the green beans.

3. Using roughly 1 tablespoon of fish mixture, form a flat, round cake; repeat until all of the mixture is used.

4. Heat roughly to ¼ inch of vegetable oil to 350 degrees on moderate to high heat in a frying pan or deep fryer; fry the fish cakes until golden.

Serve with a dipping sauce of your choice.

Yield: 15–20 small cakes

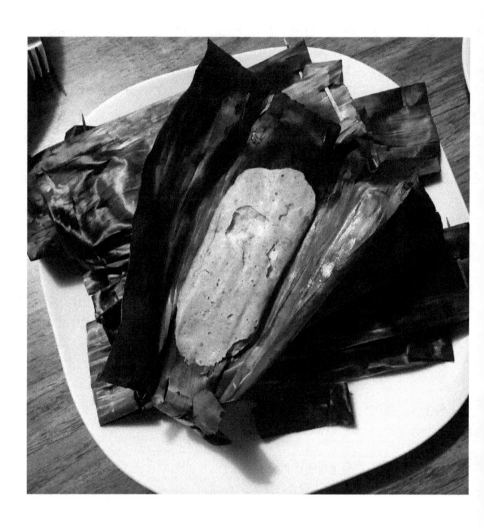

FRIED TOFU WITH DIPPING SAUCES

Ingredients:

- 1 package of tofu, cut into bite-sized cubes
- Dipping sauces of your choice Vegetable oil for frying

Directions:

1. Put in approximately two to three inches of vegetable oil to a deep fryer or wok. Heat the oil on medium until it reaches about 350 degrees. Cautiously add some of the tofu pieces, ensuring not to overcrowd them; fry until a golden-brown colour is achieved, turning continuously. Move the fried tofu to paper towels to drain as each batch is cooked.

2. Serve the tofu with a choice of dipping sauces, such as Sweet-and- Sour, Peanut, and Minty Dipping Sauce .

Yield: Servings 2–4

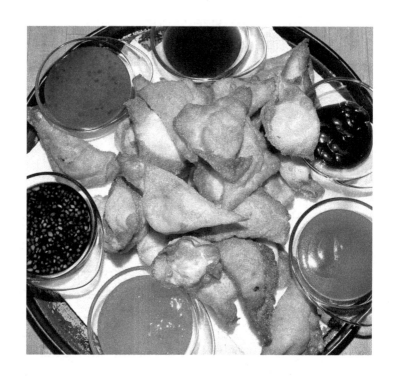

Lightning Source UK Ltd.
Milton Keynes UK
UKHW020641060521
383241UK00015B/1139